USMLE STEP 2 CK
Hematology
and
Musculoskeletal
In Your Pocket

✓ Study guide for the USMLE STEP 2 CK exam.

✓ Prepare for your shelf examination.

✓ Be ready for your inpatient rotation.

Gregory J. Fernandez M.D.

First Edition, 2016
Author & Editor: Gregory J. Fernandez, M.D.
Peer Reviewers: Urshil Kisu Patel, M.D. & Tahira N. Sánchez Muñoz, M.D.
Publisher: M.D. Educational Services
Book Design: Marie Meyer
Copyediting: Editage Cactus Communications

ISBN-13: 978-1537224572

ISBN-10: 1537224573

This book is gratefully dedicated to my wife. Thank you for your support and always being there for me. Thank you for your kindness, your devotion, and your endless selflessness support. I love you... Thank you mother, father, step-mother, brothers, friends, and family for all your encouragement and endless love. Best of luck to all the medical dreamers, the road is long and I hope my book helps you through this journey. All the best...

How to Use
"Hematology & Musculoskeletal In Your Pocket"

Hematology & Musculoskeletal In Your Pocket is a study guide for the USMLE STEP 2 CK exam that you can also use to prepare for your shelf examination and to get ready for your inpatient rotation. It is part of a series, each dealing with a different subject or sub-specialty, focusing on vital clinical knowledge.

The subjects and topics within hematology and musculosketal are called out in large, colored type. These items are also included in the Table of Contents for ease of access.

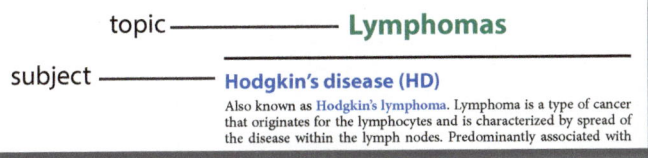

Many subjects also contain sub-subjects that are also called out in bold, blue type either as bulleted items or in-line with the text, as appropriate. They are all referenced in the index.

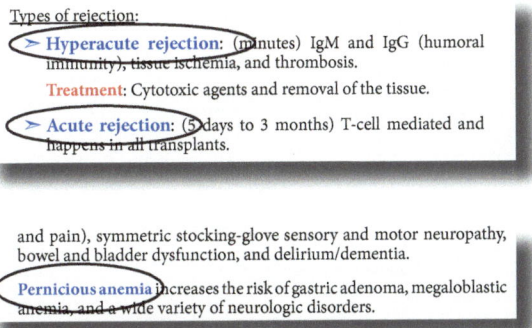

Presentation of clinical history and physical exam (Hx/PE), step-by-step diagnosis, and treatment plan are indicated by bold red headings.

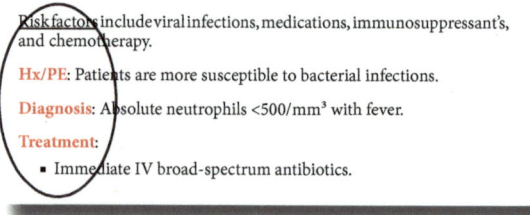

Procedures, triads, pathology, medications, antibodies and findings are called out in bold text. These items are also included in the index.

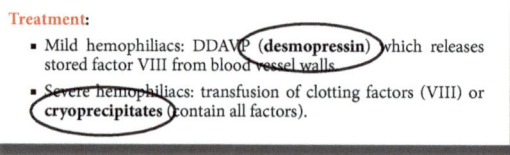

Reflexes, signs and maneuvers are shown in purple text.

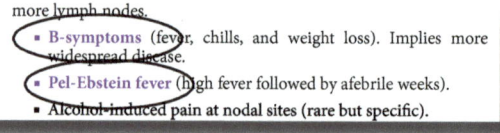

Mnemonics and key words are shown in orange text.

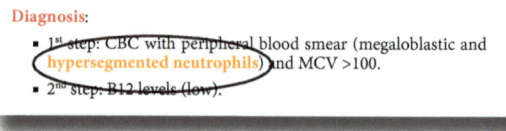

And, finally, for the avoidance of doubt, circumstances that amount to a medical emergency are flagged with a warning.

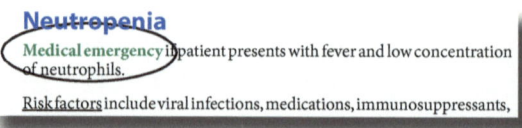

Hematology
Table of Contents

Musculoskeletal
Table of Contents

Hematology

Bleeding disorders

Hemophilia A (factor VIII deficiency)

X-linked disorder causing deficiency of clotting factor VIII, which is more common than hemophilia B. More commonly affecting men and women are usually carriers. Can be <u>hereditary</u> or <u>acquired</u> secondary to antibodies against clotting factors.

<u>Examples</u> of acquired causes are blood transfusion, postpartum, and autoimmune diseases.

Hx/PE: Hemorrhages into deep tissues and joints (hemarthrosis), arthropathy, and joint destruction.

Diagnosis:

- *First tests*, order: PT (normal), PTT (elevated), platelets (normal), and bleeding time (normal).
- Conduct a **mixing study** (normal plasma mixed with patient's plasma): corrected PTT levels after mixing study, leads to likely diagnosis of factor deficiency.
- Obtain factor assay: VII, VIII (low), IX, XI, and XII.
    - Low levels of factor VIII (<10 IU).
- Family history and genetic testing.
- *Mild* deficiency (>5% normal), *moderate* deficiency (1–5% normal), and *severe* deficiency (<1% normal).

Note:

✓ The more prolonged PTT, the more severe hemophilia.

✓ About 50% of patients transfused for hemophilia A will develop antibodies to factor VIII.

Treatment:

- *Mild hemophilia*: DDAVP (**desmopressin**) which releases stored factor VIII from blood vessel walls.

- *Severe hemophilia*: transfusion of clotting factors (VIII) or **cryoprecipitates** (contain all factors).

Note: decrease fluid intake with DDAVP medication. Desmopression retains water.

Hemophilia B (factor IX deficiency)

Also known as Christmas disease. X-linked mutation of the factor IX gene and nearly always affects men and women are usually carriers. Less common than hemophilia A.

Hx/PE: Hemorrhages into deep tissues and joints (hemarthrosis), arthropathy, and joint destruction.

Diagnosis:

- *First step*, order: PT (normal), PTT (elevated), platelets (normal), and bleeding time (normal).

- Conduct a **mixing study**: if normalized PTT levels after mixing study, most likely a factor deficiency.

- Obtain factor assay: VII, VIII, IX (low), XI, and XII.

- Family history and genetic testing.

Treatment:

- Transfusion with clotting factor (IX) or cryoprecipitates.

- DDAVP is not helpful here because not a factor VIII problem.

Note:

✓ Factor VIII has a half-life of 12 hours (dose BID).

✓ Factor IX only needs to be dosed once a day.

Hemophilia C (factor XI deficiency)

Different from hemophilia A and B, as hemophilia C has autosomal recessive inheritance and does not present with hemarthrosis. More common in Ashkenazi Jews.

Hx/PE: Bruising, nosebleeds, and heavy menstrual bleeding. No hemarthrosis.

Diagnosis:

- *First order*: PT (normal), PTT (prolonged), platelets (normal), and bleeding time (normal).
- Mixing studies: if PTT improves, more likely a clotting factor dysfunction.
- Obtain clotting factors: VII, VIII, IX, XI (low), and XII.
- Family history and genetic testing.

Treatment: Transfusion with deficient clotting factor (factor XI) or cryoprecipitates.

von Willebrand's disease (vWD)

Type 1 and type 2 are inherited as an autosomal dominant disease and is the *most common* inherited bleeding disorder. Presents with deficient or defective vWF (a protein required for platelet adhesion) and low levels of factor VIII.

Hx/PE: Easy bruising, epistaxis, oral bleeding, and menorrhagia. Joint bleeding is uncommon.

Diagnosis:

- *First order*: PT (normal), PTT (underlined: elevated), platelets (normal), and bleeding time (underlined: increased).
- Mixing studies (confirmatory test): add normal plasma to plasma and then measure PT and PTT.
- Obtain clotting factor VIII (decreased) and vWF (decreased).
- *Most accurate test*: **ristocetin cofactor assay** (capacity of vWF to agglutinate platelets).
- Family history and genetic testing.

- *Mild disease*, first line treatment is DDAVP <u>or</u> desmopressin.
- *Severe disease* or before surgery, use factor VIII concentrates, which also contains von Willebrand factors <u>or</u> cryoprecipitates.
- If menorrhagia, use OCPs and avoid aspirin.

Rule of thumb:

➤ <u>Coagulation factor disorders</u>: can cause hemarthrosis and bleeding into tissues and joints.

➤ <u>Platelet disorders</u>: can cause petechiae and easy bruising.

Coagulation medications

Warfarin

An anti-coagulant (blood thinner) that reduces the <u>formation</u> of clots. Inhibits vitamin K dependent cofactors (factors 2, 7, 9, and 10), which in turn increases PT and PTT (inhibits intrinsic and extrinsic pathways). Activated by <u>endothelium</u> (produced by tissue factor). Warfarin is teratogenic (mainly in first trimester) and hCG levels need to be obtained in reproductive women).

➤ International normalized ratio (INR) goal is usually 2.0–3.0.

➤ INR goal, if patient has a mechanical valve is 3.0–4.0.

➤ If <u>supra</u>therapeutic, stop warfarin and restart when therapeutic.

Note:

✓ If INR <5, discontinue warfarin and restart warfarin when therapeutic.

✓ If INR >5, discontinue warfarin and administer vitamin K until therapeutic.

<u>Antidote</u>: vitamin K (slow reversal) or fresh frozen plasma (FFP) (fast reversal). With FFP, match blood type for donor (example: AB blood type recuouebt with type AB donor).

Note:

✓ Warfarin inhibits proteins C and S <u>before</u> vitamin K cofactors. Beware of use in patients with renal failure.

✓ Oral vitamin K is preferred over IV vitamin K due to the reduced risk of anaphylaxis.

Warfarin-induced skin necrosis

Occurs three to five days after drug therapy is begun with warfarin. Warfarin first inhibits protein C, which can lead to pain, erythema, and full skin necrosis days after administration of warfarin. Most common sites are hip, breast, and thigh.

Treatment: Can heal spontaneously or may require surgical debridement or skin grafting.

Tissue plasminogen activator (Tpa)

A <u>clot buster</u> used with pathology such as pulmonary embolism, myocardial infarction, and strokes.

➤ Mechanism: converts plasminogen --> plasmin (chops fibrin: creating fibrin slits and D-dimer). TPa has the ability to bust clots, unlike heparin which is more suitable for clot prevention.

➤ Once factor XIII forms, TPa is not helpful. This is why there is a specific time period for TPa, as it only dissolves clots during early formation.

Heparin

Activates *anti-thrombin III*, increases PTT, inhibits intrinsic pathway only, and disrupts the conversion of fibrinogen. Activated by *collagen*. Not a clot buster, but prevents clots from forming. May cause heparin-induced thrombocytopenia (HIT) approximately 5–7 days after starting medication (especially with use of unfractionated heparin).

Administer heparin-to-warfarin conversion to decrease paradoxical hypercoagulability.

Antidote: **protamine sulfate** (dose 1mg per 100 units of heparin given over 4 hours).

Heparin-induced thrombocytopenia (HIT)

➢ A process where the immune system forms antibodies against heparin, resulting in destruction of platelets.

➢ Thrombosis is the most common clinical manifestation.

➢ More common when using unfractionated heparin than when using low molecular weight heparin (LMWH).

➢ With HIT, it is contraindicated to use LMWHs (such as enoxaparin, because it can cross-react with heparin and exacerbate thrombocytopenia.

➢ LMWH is less likely to cause HIT than unfractionated heparin.

➢ Once diagnosed with HIT need to avoid all forms of heparin from future use.

➢ It is better to substitute with argatroban (factor Xa inhibitor), lepirudin, or fondaparinux.

Diagnosis: Clinical diagnosis or **heparin factor 4 antibody**.

Treatment: *First step* is to stop heparin and use argatroban or lepirudin.

Note: safe to use fondaparinux during pregnancy.

Enoxaparin (LMWH)

➢ Inhibits Xa, dose once or twice daily, no need to monitor platelets, lower risk of HIT, and can be expensive.

➢ For patients with renal failure; unfractionated heparin is a better choice.

➢ Enoxaparin does not cross the placenta.

➢ Some medications can increase your risk of bleeding while using heparin, such as aspirin and NSAIDs.

Hypercoagulable states

Thrombophilia's or prothrombotic states. Increased risk of thromboembolic disease with <u>genetic</u> (Factor V Leiden), <u>acquired</u> (diseases and lifestyle), or <u>physiologic</u> (age, OCPs, HRT, CHF, liver disease, SLE, and pregnancy) origins.

Hx/PE: Can present with recurrent thrombotic complications such as DVT, pulmonary embolism, MI, stroke, and arterial thrombosis.

Diagnosis:

- Work-up: PTT, PT/INR, platelets, and bleeding time.
- Special tests: anti-thrombin III deficiency, factor V, proteins C and S, anti-phospholipid antibody, ANA, and homocysteine levels.

Treatment: Use heparin-to-warfarin conversion.

- 1st DVT episode: warfarin continued for 3–6 months.
- 2nd DVT episode: warfarin continued for 6–12 months.
- 3rd DVT episode: warfarin continued for lifetime.

Platelet dysfunctions

Disseminated intravascular coagulation (DIC)

Depletion of both clotting factors and platelets with deposition of fibrin in small blood vessels. Common in hospitalized patients.

<u>Risks factors</u>: associated with delivery, infection, sepsis, neoplasm, trauma, and intravascular hemolysis.

Hx/PE:

- ➤ Characteristics of both factor-type bleeding and platelet-type bleeding.
- ➤ <u>Acute</u>: bleeding from venipuncture sites, ecchymosis, and petechiae.

➤ Chronic: ecchymosis, mucosal bleeding, and thrombophlebitis (platelet and factor bleeding).

Diagnosis:

- CBC with peripheral blood smear (schistocytes/ microangiopathy), PTT (increased), PT (increased), bleeding time (increased), platelets (decreased), and D-dimers (increased).
- Elevated BUN/Cr ratio, elevated LDH, and indirect bilirubin.

Note: resembles liver disease, however, decreased factor VIII not seen in liver disease.

Treatment:

- Correct underlying causes.
- Replace clotting factors and platelets as needed (platelets <20,000).
- Corticosteroids (decrease microthrombi).
- Plasmapheresis (severe).
- Splenectomy (rarely needed).

Note: as a rule of thumb, 6 units of platelets should increase platelet count by 30,000/μL. Or 1 unit equals 5,000 μL. If does not increase, most likely secondary to antibodies against platelets.

Thrombotic thrombocytopenic purpura (TTP)

This condition can be caused by a *protease ADAMTS-13* deficiency. Platelets can cause microthrombi and small vessel ischemia. Can also lead to RBC fragmentation (hemolysis) and microangiopathic hemolytic anemia.

Hx/PE: "FATRN": fever, anemia (elevated LDH), thrombocytopenia (increased bleeding time), renal failure (ischemia), and neurological disorder (strokes). Leading to bruising and purpura. Altered mental status with TTP is more prominent than in HUS.

Note: renal failure is more severe in HUS and neurological problems are more severe in TTP.

- *First step*, order CBC with peripheral blood smears (schistocytes, platelets [low], H/H [low]), bilirubin (high), and LDH (high).
- BUN/Cr ratio: elevated.

Treatment:

- Supportive therapy or high volume plasmapheresis (*first line treatment*). Plasmapheresis replaces ADAMT-13.
- If untreated about a 95% mortality rate.

<u>Monitoring</u>: platelets and schistocytes are used to monitor disease progression or remission.

Note: do not transfuse with platelets or administer antibiotics.

Hemolytic-uremic syndrome (HUS)

Commonly triggered after a diarrheal infection with *E. coli* 0157:H7 (about 5–10 days after onset of diarrhea). Usually presents with acute renal failure, hemolytic anemia (microangiopathic hemolytic anemia), and thrombocytopenia.

Diagnosis:

- CBC with peripheral blood smear (schistocytes, platelets [low] and H/H [low]), bilirubin (high), LDH (high), and electrolytes (elevated potassium).
- BUN/Cr ratio: elevated (usually worse than in TTP).

Treatment: Supportive therapy or plasmapheresis (*first line treatment*). Children might need dialysis.

Note: with HUS, platelet transfusion and most antibiotics are contraindicated. However, quinolones may decrease the risk of hemolytic uremic syndrome.

Idiopathic thrombocytopenic purpura (ITP)

An autoimmune disease with isolated thrombocytopenia, which is more common in women. Characterized by IgG antibodies against platelets creating megakaryocytes (large platelets). Associated with lymphoma, leukemia, SLE, and human immunodeficiency virus (HIV).

Types:

➤ Acute: usually after a viral infection.

➤ Chronic: usually women 20–40 years of age and commonly unrelated to infection.

Hx/PE: Minor bleeding, easy bruising, petechiae, hematuria, and mucocutaneous bleeding.

Diagnosis:

- Diagnosis by exclusion:
  - CBC (thrombocytopenia) with peripheral blood smear (megakaryocytes).
  - **Platelet-associated antibodies** (only 80% *specific*).
  - Splenic ultrasound: usually normal spleenic size.
  - Bone marrow biopsy performed when in doubt or not treated by standard treatment: normal or megakaryocytes.

Treatment:

- Often follows an infection and spontaneously resolves within 2–6 months.
- Platelets >30,000 manage with close monitoring and usually patient is asymptomatic.
- Platelets <30,000, continued low platelets for >1 year, or bleeding, then start corticosteroids (*first line treatment*).
- IVIG (*second line therapy*) is expensive, but very <u>fast</u> way to increase platelet count; however, only lasts a few weeks.
- Anti–D (Rh factor) and rituximab might be helpful to confuse macrophages to destroy RBCs instead of platelets.
- Splenectomy if treatment fails; however, most patients will eventually need this.

Note:

✓Platelet transfusions are not recommended because the transfusions can cause antibodies against platelets. However, if severe or widespread bleeding becomes life threatening transfuse platelets.

✓ FFP not helpful because there are no platelets in FFP.

✓ If platelets >30,000 the patient is usually asymptomatic.

HELLP syndrome

Can be a life-threatening obstetrics complication that is often associated with preeclampsia and pregnancy. "HELLP": hemolysis, elevated liver enzymes, and low platelets.

Hx/PE: RUQ or epigastric abdominal pain, edema, proteinuria, headache, visual changes, elevated blood pressure, seizure, nausea, and vomiting.

Diagnosis:

- CBC (low platelets and H/H), UA (proteinuria), and elevated blood pressure.
- Elevated LDH and bilirubin levels (from hemoglobin breakdown).
- Liver enzymes (elevated AST and ALT).

Treatment:

- There is a more detailed approach in *Obstetrics in Your Pocket.*
- Deliver baby as soon as possible and always make sure mother is stable before induction.
- Anemia (administer blood transfusion), seizure prophylaxis (IV magnesium sulfate), and hypertension (IV labetalol).
- If platelets <100,000/mm^3, start IV corticosteroids and infuse platelets if <20,000/mm^3.
- DIC can be treated with fresh frozen plasma.

Viral induced thrombocytopenia

More commonly after an upper respiratory infection.

Diagnosis: CBC (platelets [low]) and increased bleeding time.

Treatment: Often self-limiting. If platelets <30,000, then consider corticosteroid administration.

Microcytic anemia

➤ *First test* to order is a CBC with peripheral blood smear (low hematocrit and hemoglobin).

➤ MCV will distinguish between microcytic, normocytic, and macrocytic anemia.

➤ Blood pressure can be a useful tool as an indicator of blood loss.

➤ All forms of anemia will present with fatigue and later become short of breath if more severe.

Iron deficiency

Microcytic iron deficiency anemia is most commonly caused by blood loss. Other causes are insufficient dietary intake, advanced growth, heavy menstruation, malnutrition, medications, and pregnancy.

Common causes:

➤ Younger patients, consider growth spurts and malnutrition.

➤ Fertile women, consider increased blood loss secondary to menstruation.

➤ Elderly patients, consider colorectal cancer.

Hx/PE: Fatigue (most common presentation), dizziness, weakness, brittle nails, pica (ice or soil craving), angular cheilitis, glossitis, SOB (*worsening* anemia), and "spoon nails." Look for pica in question stem.

Diagnosis:

- *Best initial test* is CBC (low H/H) with peripheral blood smears (hypochromic/microcytic RBCs).

- MCV (microcytic), LDH (elevated), RDW (elevated), reticulocytes (low), haptoglobin, and bilirubin (elevated).

- Order: iron (low), ferritin (low), and TIBC (high).

  - Iron studies: decreased iron and ferritin (sensitive) and increased total iron binding capacity (TIBC).

- *Most accurate test* is bone marrow biopsy (decreased reticulocytes), but test is rarely used.

- Consider colonoscopy in men or women with anemia and patients aged >50 years.

Note: low reticulocytes can be associated with worsening iron, vitamin B12, and folic acid deficiencies.

Treatment:

- Oral **iron sulfate** (4–6 weeks) can lead to constipation or diarrhea and abdominal pain.
  - Iron therapy *first* increases reticulocyte production.
  - Also, remember patient can have black stools while on iron sulfate, which is <u>not</u> blood.
  - Avoid antacids because they decrease the absorption of iron.
  - Continue iron replacement for about 8 weeks after normalizing iron levels.
- IV iron dextran (in *severe cases*), which should be administered by a hematologist.
- In infants, limit cow's milk.

Thalassemia

Hereditary, autosomal recessive, microcytic anemia, and decreased or abnormal globin chain formation. Individuals with thalassemia can have overload of iron stores from the actual disease or from transfusions.

- ➤ **α-thalassemia** (common in Africans): mutation of 1–4 α genes.
- ➤ **β-thalassemia** (common in people from the Middle East): mutation of 1–2 β genes.

Types:

- ➤ α-1: **silent**, α-2: **trait**, α-3: **H-disease**, or α-4: **hydrops fetalis**.
- ➤ **β-minor**: 1β or **β-major**: 2β.

Diagnosis:

- *Best initial test* is CBC (low H/H) with peripheral blood smear: "**target cells**."
- MCV (microcytic). Iron studies: <u>normal</u> (iron, ferritin, and TIBC).

- **Hemoglobin electrophoresis** (*most accurate test*). Test might not catch silent or trait deletions.
- DNA studies (*most specific test*) can tell you exactly how many gene deletions.

Treatment:

- β-thalassemia major and hemoglobin H disease: multiple transfusions needed.
- If *severe*: bone marrow transplant.
- Iron overload related to thalassemia may be treated with deferoxamine.

Note: α-1: silent (asymptomatic), α-2: trait (rarely needs to treat), α-3: H-disease (usually require transfusions), or α-4: hydrops fetalis (death in utero).

Sideroblastic anemia

Microcytic anemia caused by dysfunctional heme synthesis that can be inherited, acquired, or idiopathic. More frequent in alcoholics, lead poisoning, and INH usage.

Diagnosis:

- CBC (anemia) with peripheral blood smear (basophilic stippling [if lead poisoning]), MCV (microcytic), iron (increased), ferritin (high), and TIBC (normal to decreased).
- If lead toxicity:
  - Blood lead levels (elevated).
  - *Most accurate test* is **Prussian blue stain** (ringed sideroblasts).

Treatment:

- *First step* is to remove toxin and some studies show that moderate to high doses of B6 are helpful (if caused by INH).
- In *severe* cases, perform transfusions or bone marrow transplant.
- Iron overload treat with **deferoxamine**.

Anemia of chronic disease

Can cause microcytic or normocytic. Secondary to underlying disease such as rheumatic arthritis, ESRD, infection, or autoimmune diseases (SLE).

Diagnosis:

- Best initial test: CBC with peripheral blood smear.
- Iron studies: iron (low), TIBC (low), ferritin (increased), and transferrin receptor (normal).

Treatment: Treat underlying causes (e.g., rheumatic arthritis, SLE) and iron supplementation.

Megaloblastic anemia or macrocytic anemia

*Vitamin B12 and folate deficiency (both interfere with DNA Synthesis).

B12 deficiency (subacute combined degeneration)

Degeneration of many combined CNS regions. Can lead to megaloblastic anemia, peripheral neuropathy (numbness, tingling, and pain), symmetric stocking-glove sensory and motor neuropathy, bowel and bladder dysfunction, and delirium/dementia.

Pernicious anemia increases the risk of gastric adenoma, megaloblastic anemia, and a wide variety of neurologic disorders.

Risk factors: Crohn's disease, malabsorption, pernicious anemia, tapeworm, diarrhea, pancreatitis, metformin (blocks absorption), or small bowel surgery.

Diagnosis:

- *1st step*: CBC with peripheral blood smear (megaloblastic and hypersegmented neutrophils) and MCV >100.

- 2nd *step*: B12 levels (low) *most accurate test.*
- 3rd *step*: if B12 levels are normal with continued suspicion, order MMA levels (high).
- 4th *step*: **anti-intrinsic factor antibody** or **anti-parietal cell antibodies** (*specific* for pernicious anemia).
- Blood smear is an important finding and helps confirm), as B12 levels can be a false positive.

Note: **Schilling test** has been largely replaced by **anti-parietal cell antibodies** (pernicious anemia). However, Schilling's test works as follows:

✓ Inject IM B12 unlabeled <u>plus</u> oral radiolabeled B12. If excreted in urine, then dietary insufficiency.

✓ If B12 not in urine, administer intrinsic factor and radiolabeled oral B12. If in urine, then diagnose pernicious anemia.

✓ If B12 still not in urine, likely *Diphyllobothrium latum.*

Treatment:
- Secondary to <u>malnutrition</u>: administer oral or IM vitamin B12.
- Secondary to <u>pernicious anemia</u>: administer intrinsic factor and oral B12.
- Secondary to *Ascaris lumbricoides*: administer mebendazole, which is the treatment of choice.

Note: monitor potassium when infusing vitamin B12, to prevent hypokalemia.

Folic acid

Megaloblastic anemia can be caused by decreased dietary folate, malabsorption, alcoholism, pregnancy, SMP-TMX, MTX, and drugs (inhibit DNA synthesis). <u>No</u> neurological signs with folic acid.

Hx/PE: Fatigue, pallor, and weakness.

Diagnosis:
- 1st *step*: CBC with peripheral blood smear (megaloblastic and hypersegmented neutrophils) and MCV >100.

- *2nd step*: measure B12 and folic acid levels (low). Folic acid levels is the *most accurate test*.

- *3rd step*: measure MMA and homocysteine levels, if normal folic acid levels with continued suspicion:
  - Both MMA and homocysteine are elevated in B12 deficiency.
  - Normal MMA and elevated homocysteine are present in folic acid deficiency.

- Bone marrow biopsy: rarely performed.

Treatment: Treat underlying cause and problematic medications. Administer (oral, IM or IV) B12 and folic acid.

Normocytic anemia

*Bone marrow unable to compensate for increased RBC damage or hypoproliferative states. All will have elevated bilirubin levels, elevated LDH, and low H/H.

Sickle cell disease (SCD)

Autosomal recessive, normocytic anemia, defective β-globin chain at the 6th position (substitution of glutamate for valine). Increased RBC destruction and vaso-occlusion; usually appears after 6 months of age because of Hbg-F protection in infants.

Hx/PE: Jaundice, cholelithiasis, delayed growth, pneumococcal infections, infarction, vaso-occlusion (ischemic organ damage), splenic infarction, painful crises, infections, urinary tract infection, dehydration, splenic sequestration crises (high risk, especially in children), aplastic crisis (B19 virus), and osteomyelitis (*staphylococcus aureus* and *salmonella*).

Diagnosis:
- CBC (decreased H/H), MCV (80–100), and reticulocytes (low).
- Blood smear: "sickle cell shape" (seen in disease not trait) or target cells.

- Aplastic crisis: transient low hemoglobin and reticulocytes.
- *Most accurate test* is **hemoglobin electrophoresis** (*gold standard*).

Treatment:

- **Vaso-occlusion crisis**: *first step* is pain control <u>followed</u> by hydration (use 1/2 normal saline if normal blood pressure, and normal saline if hypotensive), oxygen, and antibiotics (if fever and/or lymphocytosis).
  - Diphenhydramine helps control itching associated with the use of opioids.
- If develops fever and elevated WBCs (start IV ceftriaxone and levofloxacin immediately), can become septic quickly do <u>not</u> wait until labs to return.
- If painful crisis >4 times per year, use **hydroxyurea** (<u>decreases</u> frequency and severity of pain crisis).
- Folic acid supplementation in these patients is helpful (1 mg dose of folic acid daily for life).
- Penicillin daily prophylaxis from birth to five years of age.
- IVIGs and transfusion might be the only treatment for B19 aplastic crisis.
- If *severe*: transfusions or bone marrow transplants (the only known cure for SCD).
- Last resort: splenectomy.
  - If **splenic sequestration** (will need prophylactic vaccinations). More common in children.
- Asplenic patients that present with fever or lymphocytosis will need to be started on vancomycin and ceftriaxone.
- Genetic counseling before partners have a child.

<u>Prophylaxis vaccinations</u>: pneumonia and *Haemophilus influenzae*.

Note: sudden drop in hematocrit, consider parvovirus B19.

Glucose-6-phosphate dehydrogenase deficiency (G6PD)

Causes spontaneous destruction of RBC (hemolysis). G6PD is an enzyme in the *pentose phosphate pathway*. An X-linked recessive genetic diseases that causes oxidative stress, which leads to "bite cells," "Heinz bodies," and increased RBC destruction.

Risk factors: males, infection, intake of fava beans, oxidative stress, sulfonamides, and anti-malarial therapy.

Diagnosis:

- *Best initial test*: CBC with blood smear (showing **Heinz bodies** [denatured oxidized hemoglobin]).
- Electrolytes, MCV (normal), LDH (elevated), and bilirubin levels (elevated).
- Test **G6PD** levels (months after episodes, as can be normal during episodes) and genetic testing.

Treatment: Take away stressors and consider transfusions or splenectomy (rarely).

Note: reticulocyte count helps determine if secondary to RBC destruction or hypoproliferative states.

✓ RBC destruction will have elevated reticulocyte count.

✓ Hypoproliferative states will have low reticulocyte count.

Paroxysmal nocturnal hemoglobinuria (PNH)

Increased complement system activation (intrinsic immune system) and destruction of RBCs. Defect in *phosphatidylinositol glycan A*, which causes no protection on the RBC membrane. Cause of death is usually large vessel venous thrombosis (example, portal vein thrombosis) in about 40% of patients.

Hx/PE: Reddish colored urine, SOB, fatigue, and dizziness.

- *Best initial test* is **sugar test**, CBC (anemia), LDH (increased), UA (best to measure in the morning), and reticulocytes (elevated).
- *Most accurate test*: **flow cytometry**, demonstrating deficiency of CD55 or CD59 on RBCs.

Treatment:

- *Best initial treatment* is corticosteroids and iron. Consider transfusions in severe cases of anemia.
- Warfarin decreases the risk of thrombosis.

Hereditary spherocytosis

Autosomal dominant and characterized by RBC membrane destruction from abnormal spectrin and/or ankyrin production causing splenic destruction. RBCs are sphere-shaped, rather than bi-concave circular shaped.

Diagnosis:

- CBC with peripheral blood smear (spherocytes), Coombs test (negative), and genetic testing.
- *Most accurate test*: **osmolarity fragility test**.

Treatment: Folic acid supplementation and splenectomy.

Note: in both hereditary spherocytosis and sickle cell anemia, folic acid is useful.

Autoimmune RBC destruction

Autoimmune destruction of RBCs that can be exacerbated by EBV, chronic lymphocytic leukemia (CLL), mycoplasma, and medications (penicillin, alpha-methyldopa, and sulfa drugs).

Diagnosis:

- CBC with peripheral blood smear, LDH, and bilirubin.

- *Most accurate diagnostic test*: **Coombs test** (positive).
  - Coombs test is positive for IgG (warm).
  - Coombs test is negative for IgM (cold).

Treatment:

- *Best initial therapy*: steroids (prednisone) and transfusion (if needed).
- IVIGs (not definitive treatment but stops the destruction of RBC, fast) is used once steroids and transfusions have failed.
- When above fails, consider splenectomy.

Aplastic anemia

Destruction of bone marrow cells causing pancytopenia (anemia, leukopenia, and thrombocytopenia) which can be caused by Fanconi's anemia, autoimmune disease, radiation, benzene, HIV, EBV, and toxins.

➤ Fanconi's syndrome: café au lait spots, short stature, and radial/thumb hypoplasia aplasia.

Hx/PE: Pancytopenia: pallor, fatigue, weakness, petechiae, bruising, bleeding, and infection.

Diagnosis:

- CBC with peripheral blood smear: H/H (decreased), platelets (decreased), and WBC (decreased). Decrease in all three lines.
- MCV (increased to normal).
- *Most accurate test*: bone marrow biopsy shows predominance of fat and stroma with cellular hypoplasia.

Treatment:

- ➤ Younger than 50 years of age: treat underlying infections, platelet transfusions, blood transfusions, and bone marrow transplantation (potential cure).
- ➤ Older than 50 years of age: treat underlying infections and cyclosporine (immunosuppressant).

Microangiopathic hemolytic anemia (MHA)

Destruction of red blood cells that can be precipitated by TTP, HUS, and DIC.

Diagnosis: CBC with peripheral blood smear (schistocytes), LDH (elevated), bilirubin (elevated), and D-dimers (elevated).

Treatment: Treat underlying causes: TTP and HUS (plasmapheresis), and DIC (correct underlying causes).

Note: for TTP and HUS, do <u>not</u> administer platelets, antibiotics, or steroids.

Mechanical hemolysis

Can be seen in patients with mechanical heart valves.

Hx/PE: Pallor, fatigue, tachycardia, tachypnea, and jaundice.

Diagnosis: CBC (low H/H) with blood smear (schistocytes), reticulocytes (high), LDH (high), and bilirubin (high).

Polycythemias

Polycythemias

An abnormal elevation of RBCs out of proportion to the blood volume that can be either primary or secondary.

➤ Primary polycythemia (also known as polycythemia vera).
A dysfunction of the bone marrow that causes an abnormal increase in RBCs and often increases in all three-cell lines.

Hx/PE: Hyperviscosity syndrome (thick blood) which can lead to hypertension, hepatosplenomegaly, decreased tissue blood flow, and oxygenation. Presents with flushing, sweating, pruritus after hot bath, hypoxia, and increased risk of transient ischemic attack (TIA).

Diagnosis:

- *Initial test*: CBC: commonly has an <u>increase</u> in all three-cell lines (WBCs, RBCs, and platelets).
- Measure erythropoietin (low, because of negative feedback).
- Arterial blood gas (ABG): access hypoxia.
- *More accurate test* is **JAK2 mutation** (97% sensitive) and seen in 95% of the cases.

Treatment:

- *Best initial test* is phlebotomy: maintain hematocrit <45% in men and <42% in women.
- Aspirin: prevents thrombosis.
- Add **hydroxyurea** as adjuvant treatment if >70 years old, thrombotic events, platelet count >1,500,000/mm^3, or cardiovascular risk factors.

➤ **Secondary polycythemia**: increased hematocrit and increased erythropoietin secondary to hypoxia, smoking, chronic obstructive pulmonary disease (COPD), sleep apnea, high altitudes, decreased plasma volumes, or hemoconcentration (diuresis, diarrhea, vomiting, or burns).

Diagnosis: *First step*: CBC (elevated H/H) and <u>elevated</u> erythropoietin.

Treatment: Treat underlying cause and give oxygen and fluids.

<u>Basically</u>:

- <u>Primary polycythemia</u>: increased hematocrit with decreased erythropoietin levels.
- <u>Secondary polycythemia</u>: increased or normal hematocrit with increased erythropoietin levels.

Note: **neonatal polycythemia**: defined as hematocrit >65% and requires adequate hydration and partial exchange transfusion.

Porphyria cutanea tarda (PCT)

Autosomal dominant, defect in **uroporphyrinogen decarboxylase**, and abnormalities of heme production.

Associated with alcohol use, hepatitis C, hemochromatosis, barbiturates, OCPs, and fasting.

Hx/PE: Photodermatitis, skin erythema, painless blisters, neuropsychiatric symptoms, abdominal pain, seizures, and pink/brown urine.

Diagnosis: Porphyrins (blood, urine, and stool).

Treatment:

- *First step* avoid triggers: alcohol, barbiturates, OCPs, fasting, and excess exposure to sunlight.
- If *mild*: high glucose.
- If *severe*: IV hematin.
- Low does chloroquine or hydroxychloroquine can be helpful.

Leukemias

* Malignant proliferation of hematopoietic cells.

Acute lymphocytic leukemia (ALL)

This is the most common childhood malignancy. Has increased growth of immature blood cells (lymphoblasts), in which lymphoblast's are over produced in the bone marrow. Highly associated with Down's syndrome. Look for **terminal deoxynucleotidyl transferase** (TdT) and **common acute lymphocytic leukemia antigen** (CALLA) in question stem.

Hx/PE: Anemia (pallor and fatigue), thrombocytopenia (petechiae and bruising), and leukocytosis (increased infection secondary to dysfunctional WBCs). Hepatosplenomegaly with possible testicular and central nervous system (CNS) involvement.

Diagnosis:

- *Best initial test*: CBC with peripheral blood smear (WBCs [increased, decreased, or normal], H/H [low], and platelets [low]).

- Blood smear: increased blast cells >25%.
- Usually, a higher WBC equals a worse prognosis.
- Immunohistochemical testing: TdT and CALLA antigens can be helpful.
- *Most accurate test* is bone marrow biopsy.

Note: if WBC >100,000, **leukostasis,** which can cause obstruction of microcirculation.

Treatment:
- Prior to treatment, need a full work-up and physical examination.
- Treatment includes controlling infections, administration of transfusion, and bone marrow transplants (severe).
- *Best treatment*: chemotherapy and radiation (98% cure rate).
  - Maintain chemotherapy for 2–3 years after remission.
- Patient can develop meningeal leukemia: *best agent* to treat is intrathecal methotrexate.

Note: prior to chemotherapy, use allopurinol to prevent hyperuricemia and hydrate patient.

Acute myeloid leukemia (AML)

A cancer of the myeloid blood cells that cause an increase in myeloblasts and more common in adults. Elevated M3 is associated with **auer rods** (eosinophilic needle-shaped inclusions), and DIC (risk of strokes and myocardial infarction).

Diagnosis:
- *First step*: CBC with peripheral blood smear: WBC (increased, decreased, or normal), H/H (low), and platelets (low).
  - Blood smear: increased myeloblasts and "auer rods."
- Myeloperoxidase: positive.
- *Most accurate test* is bone marrow biopsy.

- Treat underlying infections and anemia with transfusions and bone marrow transplants (severe).
- **Acute promyelocytic leukemia (APL) t15:17**: treat with all-trans-retinoic acid therapy in addition to chemotherapy.
- Chemotherapy and radiation.

Note: prior to chemotherapy, use allopurinol and hydration to prevent hyperuricemia.

Chronic lymphocytic leukemia (CLL)

A slow-growing cancer, which begins in the lymphocytes of the bone marrow and extends into the blood. More common in older men (>50 years of age). Functionally incompetent lymphocytes in bone marrow and periphery. Associated with SLL and well-differentiated B-lymphocytes.

Hx/PE: Fatigue, malaise, infection, lymphadenopathy, and splenomegaly.

Diagnosis:

- *Best initial test*: CBC with peripheral blood smear: WBC (increased), H/H (low), and platelets (low).
  - Blood smear: "smudge cells" (are ruptured nuclei).
- Flow cytometry: CD5, CD20, CD21.
- *Most accurate test* is bone marrow biopsy, but rarely performed.

Treatment:

- Not curable, treat symptoms, and mainly palliative.
- Consider transfusions and bone marrow transplants.
- Early stages (0–1) in which there are mainly enlarged nodes and lymphocytosis:
  - No treatment is indicated.
- Later stages (2, 3, or 4), usually presents with splenomegaly, anemia, and thrombocytopenia:

- Treatment with fludarabine, cyclophosphamide, and rituximab (also known as "FCR").
- Splenectomy can be helpful for anemia and thrombocytopenia.

Chronic myeloid leukemia (CML)

Can lead to myeloid progenitor cells, which leads to leukocytosis with possible erythrocytes and elevated platelets. **BCR-ABL translocation** must be present and **Philadelphia chromosome t(9:22)** present in 95% of patients.

Accelerated disease: transition toward **blast crisis** leads to increased bone marrow and peripheral blood counts (>20% myeloblasts or lymphoblasts in the blood or bone marrow). Blasts resemble acute leukemia. Smoking can accelerate progression to blast crises.

Hx/PE: Anemia, splenomegaly (left upper quadrant pain), and hepatomegaly. **B symptoms**: fever, chills, and weight loss.

Diagnosis:

- *First test*: CBC with very high WBC, often >100,000 (leukemoid reaction, if leukocytosis >50,000), H/H (low), and platelets (low).
- *Most accurate test* is cytogenetic analysis: (Philadelphia chromosome) almost definitive diagnosis.
- Leukocyte alkaline phosphatase (LAP) is low.

Treatment:

- If young patient: consider stem cell transplant.
- *Best initial test*: imatinib (Gleevec), which inhibits BCR-ABL tyrosine kinase.
- Blast crisis: dasatinib plus hematopoietic stem cell transplant.
- The only curative treatment for CML is a bone marrow transplant or allogeneic stem cell transplant.

Note: progestins (megestrol acetate and medroxyprogesterone acetate). Best way to increase appetite in advanced cancer. Medication can cause delirium, hyperthermia, mydriasis, and urinary retention.

Hairy cell leukemia

Malignant B-lymphocytes that accumulate in the bone marrow. More commonly found in elderly individuals. Similar to CLL, except <u>rarely</u> lymphadenopathy.

Hx/PE: Anemia (fatigue, shortness of breath), thrombocytopenia (petechiae, bruising), and lymphocytopenia (infections).

Diagnosis:

- CBC with peripheral blood smear: <u>low</u> (WBC, H/H, and platelets). Resembles aplastic anemia.
    - Peripheral blood smear (hair cells or mononuclear cells with abundant pale cytoplasm and cytoplasmic projections).
- **Tartrate-resistant acid phosphatase** (**TRAP**): staining for hairy cells.
- Most patients require a bone marrow biopsy for final diagnosis.

Treatment:

- *Best initial treatment* (first-line) is **cladribine** (purine nucleoside analog).
- Might become pancytopenic: may need red blood cells and platelet transfusions.
- IFN-α (immune system hormone) helpful to few people.
- Bone marrow transplants.
- Splenectomy (severe).

Note: cladribine treats almost 95% of patients.

Leukostasis syndrome

Increased leukocytes (>100,000). Occludes microcirculation causing local hypoxemia.

Treatment: Hydroxyurea +/- **leukapheresis**.

Tumor lysis syndrome

Most commonly caused after chemotherapy treatment of lymphomas or leukemias. Causes hyperuricemia, hyperkalemia, hyperphosphatemia, and hypocalcaemia.

Treatment: Allopurinol or rasburicase and IV hydration.

Note: in tumor lysis syndrome, EKG may show prolonged QT-intervals (hypocalcaemia).

Lymphomas

Hodgkin's disease (HD)

Also known as Hodgkin's lymphoma. Lymphoma is a type of cancer that originates for the lymphocytes and is characterized by spread of the disease within the lymph nodes. Predominantly associated with EBV, bimodal age, male gender, and above diaphragm. Can present with cervical lymphadenopathy or a mediastinal mass. HD is usually found at stage I or II and usually found around the neck area.

Types:
- Nodular sclerosing (more common in women).
- Mixed cellularity.
- Lymphocyte predominance (better prognosis).
- Lymphocyte depletion (worse prognosis).

Hx/PE: The most common symptom is painless enlargement of one or more lymph nodes.
- B-symptoms (fever, chills, and weight loss). Implies more widespread disease.
- Pel-Ebstein fever (high fever followed by afebrile weeks).
- Alcohol-induced pain at nodal sites (rare but specific).

Diagnosis:
- CBC with differentials (look at lymphocytic depletion or predominance).

- Chest radiography: likely mediastinal masses.
- *Best initial test* is <u>excisional</u> lymph node biopsy: (gold standard) "Reed Sternberg cells" (bi-lobar nuclei) CD-15 and CD-30.
  - Fine needle aspiration (FNA) is not specific enough.
- Severity is based on crossing of the diaphragm, number of nodes involved, and B symptoms.

Note:
- For lymphomas, biopsy the lymph nodes.
- For leukemia's, biopsy the bone marrow.

Treatment:
- Chemotherapy:
  - "ABVD" (<u>A</u>driamycin, <u>b</u>leomycin, <u>v</u>inblastine, and <u>d</u>acarbazine).
  - "MOPP" (<u>m</u>echlorethamine, <u>O</u>ncovin [vincristine], <u>p</u>rocarbazine, and <u>p</u>rednisone).
- <u>Plus</u> radiation therapy.

Note: radiation to the neck, monitor the patient for the induction of secondary hypothyroidism.

Non-Hodgkin's lymphoma (NHL)

A type of cancer derived from lymphocytes that can be associated with HIV, diabetes mellitus, and immunosuppression. Most are of B-cell origin, but can be related with T-cells or natural killer cells. NHL is usually found in stages III and IV. Cancers are usually <u>non</u>-painful. Burkitt's has a worse prognosis.

Hx/PE: Fever, chills, painless lymphadenopathy, and weight loss.

Diagnosis:
- CBC is usually normal (which makes it different from leukemias).
- *Most accurate test* is excisional lymph node biopsy, which is needed for diagnosis (not FNA).

- Staging (typical staging includes chest, abdominal, and pelvic CT scan).
- **Ann Arbor classification**: number of nodes and if crosses the diaphragm.
- If patient is HIV positive, examine CSF if there are neurologic signs.
- Staging:
  - Stage I: one lymph node.
  - Stage II: two lymph nodes on same side of diaphragm.
  - Stage III: both sides of diaphragm.
  - Stage IV: widespread disease.

Treatment:
  - "CHOP regimen" (cyclophosphamide, hydroxydoxorubicin [Adriamycin], Oncovin [vincristine], and prednisone).
  - Stages I and II: use radiation and mild chemotherapy.
  - Stages III and IV: use chemotherapy.

Medication side effects: cyclophosphamide (hemorrhagic cystitis and bladder carcinoma), Adriamycin (cardiac toxicity), vincristine (peripheral neuropathy), vinblastine (peripheral neuropathy), bleomycin (lung fibrosis), cisplatin (ototoxicity and renal toxicity), doxorubicin (cardiomyopathy), and prednisone (osteoporosis and cataracts).

Myelomas

Multiple myeloma (MM)

A collection of abnormally high plasma cell accumulation in the bone marrow, which leads to abnormal cell growth within the bone marrow. Plasma cells (produce antibodies), which cause elevated IgG and IgA levels. Excessive production of monoclonal immunoglobulins or immunoglobulin fragments (kappa/lambda light chains). MM is the most common malignant bone tumor and more common in elderly patients. Hyperviscosity is more common in Waldenstrom's macroglobulinemia but can also happen with MM.

Triad: plasma cells (>10%), M proteins (serum or urine), and bone lytic lesions.

Monoclonal gammopathy of undetermined significance (MGUS): No renal dysfunction, no lytic lesions, plasma cells <10%, and no increase in calcium. In patients diagnosed with **MGUS** (premalignancy), close follow-up with immunoglobulin levels every 6 months for 2 years is recommended. No treatment needed; just monitor.

Rick factors: petroleum, radiation, pesticides, and other chemicals.

Hx/PE: The most common symptom is bone pain. Might develop anemia, increased uric acid, hypercalcemia, lytic bone lesions, renal abnormalities, and infections.

Tumor can cause spinal cord compression, which causes motor and sensory loss, weakness, numbness, and loss of bowel and bladder function (requires emergency surgical decompression).

Diagnosis:

- CBC with peripheral blood smear: (anemia), uric acid (elevated), electrolytes (increased calcium), BUN/Cr ratio ([elevated] secondary to calcium, and BJ proteins).
  - Blood smear: "rouleaux formations" (IgG sticks to RBCs and causes RBCs to stick together).
- *Best initial study*: skeletal survey (radiography) showing bone lytic lesions.
  - MRI more *specific* than skeletal survey.
- **Protein electrophoresis** (urine and serum):
  - Serum electrophoresis: will show elevated IgG (60%) and IgA (25%).
  - Urine electrophoresis: will show BJ proteins. BJ proteins are not seen on urinalysis.
- Bone marrow biopsy (*most specific test*): >10% plasma cells.

Note: **beta-2 microglobulin** is used as a prognostic factor and to monitor the progression of the disease.

Treatment:

- If < 70 years of age: high dose chemotherapy (melphalan) and stem cell transplant.
- If > 70 years of age: if cannot tolerate stem cell transplant consider **melphalan** and steroids.
- Hypercalcemia (hydrate and diuresis), renal failure (hydration), infection (antibiotics), bone fractures (bisphosphonates), and vaccinations (influenza and pneumonia).
- Chemotherapy but often becomes resistant by **MDR gene mutation.**
- If develop DVT, will need heparin.

Waldenstrom's macroglobulinemia (WM)

➤ B-cells leading to malignant monoclonal gammopathy. The main attributing antibody is IgM.

➤ Elevated monoclonal IgM spike can lead to hyperviscosity syndrome.

Risks: MGUS can be a precursor to both Waldenstrom's macroglobulinemia and MM.

Hx/PE: Blurred vision, AMS, headache, mucosal bleeding, vertigo, lethargy, and engorged blood vessels.

Diagnosis:

- CBC (anemia, low platelets, and low lymphocytes), electrolytes (normal calcium levels), and creatinine is occasionally elevated. Plasma viscosity (elevated) must be measured.
- Elevated: ESR, LDH, uric acid, and alkaline phosphatase.
- Serum and urine protein electrophoresis (elevated IgM).
- Bone marrow biopsy (*gold standard* and required for diagnosis), abnormal plasma cells, and **Ditcher bodies** (PAS + IgM deposits around the nucleus).

Treatment:

- *Best initial treatment* for hyperviscosity is IV fluids and plasmapheresis (removes excessive immunoglobulin).

- Added treatment: cyclophosphamide and rituximab.
- The FDA approved **ibrutinib** for use of WM in 2015.

Amyloidosis

Extracellular deposition of protein fibrils caused by buildup of misfolded proteins. Can deposit in multiple organs.

➤ **Primary amyloidosis** (AL): MM and Waldenstrom's macroglobulinemia.

➤ **Secondary amyloidosis** (AA): caused be chronic inflammation, infection, and neoplasm.

➤ Dialysis-related: B2-microglobulin deposits secondary to long-term dialysis.

➤ Alzheimer's disease: limited to one organ (brain).

Diagnosis: Requires tissue biopsy (**Congo red staining** showing "**apple-green birefringence**").

Treatment:

- Primary amyloidosis: melphalan and steroids followed by stem cell transplantation.
- Secondary amyloidosis: treat secondary condition (infection, neoplasm, or inflammation).

White blood cell disorders

Eosinophilia

Esinophiles > 4.5×10^8/L. **Absolute eosinophil count** = WBC × % eosinophils × 0.01 (normal levels do not exceed 500 cells/mcL).

Triggered by: IgE mediates eosinophil production, which is induced by basophils and mast cells. Also involved: IL-3, IL-5, and GM-CSF.

Causes: "NAACP": neoplasm, asthma, allergies (IgE), collagen vascular disease (polyarteritis nodosa [PAN], Churg-Strauss syndrome, and dermatomyositis), parasites (travel), and drugs (sulfonamides, ASA, and phenytoin).

Diagnosis:

- CBC with differential (eosinophilia).
- If headache: possible coccidioidomycosis; CSF sample.
- If hematuria: possible schistosomiasis.

Treatment: Treat underlying cause. Idiopathic eosinophilia, controlled with corticosteroids.

Neutropenia

Medical emergency if patient presents with fever and low concentration of neutrophils.

Risk factors include viral infections, medications, immunosuppressant's, and chemotherapy.

Hx/PE: Patients are more susceptible to bacterial infections.

Diagnosis: Absolute neutrophils $<500/\text{mm}^3$ with fever.

Treatment:

- Immediate IV broad-spectrum antibiotics.
- Treated with granulocyte-colony stimulating factor (G-CSF) <u>or</u> granulocyte-macrophage colony-stimulating factor (GM-CSF).

Transfusion reactions

Precautions:

- If massive transfusion: warm blood to decrease hypothermia.
- Cross matching: prevents <u>acute</u> hemolytic reaction.
- Leukoreduction: can prevent <u>non</u>-hemolytic febrile reaction.
- Cross matching blood is most difficult with patients with multiple transfusions that can create alloantibodies.

Treatment: Administer acetaminophen (Tylenol) and diphenhydramine, which can help prevent transfusion reaction.

Non-hemolytic febrile reaction

Most common type of transfusion reaction with symptoms usually within 1–6 hours.

Hx/PE: Fever, chills, tachycardia, hypotension, anemia, hemoglobinuria, and malaise.

Diagnosis: Clinical impression.

Treatment:
- Stop transfusion (*first step*), IV fluids, and diuresis.
- Acetaminophen can be used for fever.
- *Severe* cases: sodium bicarbonate to alkalinize the urine.

Prevention: leukoreduction before transfusion.

Minor allergic reaction

Hx/PE: Urticarial, hives, fever, chills, and rash.

Diagnosis: Clinical impression.

Treatment: Stop transfusion, administer anti-histamines, and administer epinephrine +/- steroids (if becomes *severe*).

Hemolytic transfusion reaction

A type of transfusion reaction associated with hemolysis and can be caused secondary to ABO mismatch.

Hx/PE: Fever, chills, tachycardia, tachypnea, and hypotension. Burning at IV site.

Diagnosis: Clinical impression.

Treatment: Stop transfusion and administer aggressive IV fluids with diuretics to increase renal blood flow. Pressors might be needed.

Prevention: cross-matching.

Transplant

Types of transplants:
- Autologous (self).
- Syngeneic (twin).
- Allogeneic (donor).

Allogeneic and syngeneic donors: check for ABO and HLA match. Organ donors need to be kept normotensive and normothermic.

Rejection reaction

An immune system response that destroys the transplanted tissue.

Types of rejection:
- **Hyperacute rejection**: (minutes) IgM and IgG (humoral immunity), tissue ischemia, and thrombosis.
  Treatment: Cytotoxic agents and removal of the tissue.

- **Acute rejection**: (5 days to 3 months) T-cell mediated and happens in all transplants.
  Diagnosis: Increased liver enzymes, alkaline phosphatase, BUN/Cr ratio, and LDH.

  Treatment: Corticosteroids, OKT3, and tacrolimus.

- **Chronic rejection**: (months to years) T-cell mediated, fibrosis, and gradual loss of organ function.
  Treatment: No treatment.

Neoplasms and associations

➤ **Ulcerative colitis** → colorectal cancer.

➤ **Cirrhosis** → hepatocellular carcinoma.

➤ **Plummer-Vinson syndrome** → squamous cell carcinoma of esophagus.

➤ **Barrett's esophagus** → esophageal adenocarcinoma.

➤ **Actinic keratosis** → squamous cell carcinoma of skin.

➤ **Tuberous sclerosis** → astrocytoma and cardiac rhabdomyoma.

➤ **Down's syndrome** → ALL.

➤ **Xeroderma pigmentosum** → squamous cell and basal cell carcinomas.

➤ **Pernicious anemia** → gastric adenocarcinoma.

➤ **Paget's disease** → osteosarcoma and RB.

➤ **Immunodeficiency** → lymphomas.

➤ **AIDS** → NHL and Kaposi's sarcoma.

➤ **Autoimmune disease** → thymomas.

➤ **Acanthosis nigricans** → visceral malignancy.

➤ **Dysplastic nevus** → malignant melanoma.

Musculoskeletal

Rheumatology

Rheumatoid arthritis (RA)

A chronic systemic autoimmune disorder that is more common in women >50 years. It is a "symmetric inflammatory" disease that involves both large and small joints and ultimately leads to erosion of tendons, cartilage, and bone. The sacroiliac joint is spared.

Risk factors: viral infections, genetic causes, HLA-DR3, HLA- DR4, and female gender.

Other presentations associated with RA:

➤ Felty's syndrome: RA, splenomegaly, and neutropenia.

➤ Atlantoaxial subluxation: involves C1 and C2 (intubation risks).

➤ Sjogren's syndrome: RA and keratoconjunctivitis sicca.

➤ Baker's cyst: popliteal mass (posterior herniation of knee synovium).

➤ Kaplan syndrome: RA and restrictive lung disease.

➤ Anemia of chronic disease: ferritin (high), TIBC (low), and iron (low).

Hx/PE: History of at least 6 weeks of painful morning stiffness that lasts >1 hour, fever, swelling, and weight loss. Involves PIP joints and rarely DIP joints.

Diagnosis:

- Primarily a clinical diagnosis (if negative rheumatoid factor and continued high clinical suspicion of RA then this is still a likely diagnosis, as rheumatoid factor levels can be negative in about 20% of patients).

- Elevated levels of ESR and CBC (elevated WBC).

- Iron studies: may show anemia of chronic disease.

- Rheumatic factor (IgM antibodies against Fc IgG): not the absolute marker for a positive diagnosis, since this factor is present in about 80% of all individuals.

- *Most accurate test*: anti-cyclic citrullinated peptide (anti-CCP).

- Synovial fluid aspiration: WBCs (3,000–50,000 cell/µL) show decreased viscosity. If very high cell count, RA needs to be considered.

- Joint radiography:

  - Early signs: swelling.

  - Late signs: joint narrowing, erosion, and "pannus formations."

Treatment:

- NSAIDs (mild cases)—*first line*.

  - This medication does not delay the progression of RA.

- The *next* medication choice for *moderate* to *severe* cases are disease-modifying anti-rheumatic drugs [DMARDs] such as methotrexate (MTX) + folic acid (**leucovorin** is a *more potent* form of folic acid).

  - Observation of bone erosion on x-ray is an indication to start MTX.

  - Folic acid helps prevent megaloblastic anemia.

- If MTX does not work alone or produces little response, then anti-TNF agents (infliximab or etanercept) will need to be added.

- Steroids are administered for *acute* inflammation and can be used as a bridge for MTX, as this medication will take time to become effective.

- Sulfasalazine and hydroxychloroquine (when conservative treatments fail).

Note:

✓ DMARD (MTX) can help delay disease progression.

✓ Viral arthritis (parvovirus) is usually self-limiting and usually only lasts a few days.

Medication side effects:

- NSAIDs (<u>inhibit</u> COX-1, which decreases levels of platelet thromboxane A2): acute renal failure, gastric ulcers (lowers prostaglandins), and drug-induced hepatitis.

- MTX: megaloblastic anemia (folic acid deficiency), elevated LFT levels (decreases with folic acid treatment), and oral ulcers.

- Hydroxychloroquine: retinopathy (dilated eye exam required yearly).

- Infliximab: need to test for tuberculosis (PPD) before use.

Osteoarthritis

Most common joint abnormality. Chronic <u>non</u>-inflammatory arthritis of the synovial joints that can involve **Bouchard's nodes** (PIP joints) and **Heberden's nodes** (DIP joints). Can involve the hands, feet, knees, hips, spine, and shoulders.

<u>Risk factors</u>: advanced age, overuse of joints, obesity, and joint trauma.

Hx/PE: Usually observed in elderly patients; involving the wear and tear of joints and morning stiffness that usually lasting <30 minutes. Pain is aggravated with activity and is worsened at the end of the day but improves with rest. Some patients present with "joint crepitus" and decreased joint movement.

Diagnosis:

- CBC (normal), ESR (normal), antinuclear antibodies (ANA) (normal), RF (normal), and anti-CCP (normal).

- *Best initial test*: joint radiography: "osteophytes" and decreased joint space.

- Synovial fluid: "straw-colored" fluid, normal viscosity, and WBC count <2,000 cells/μL (low).

Treatment:

- Weight loss and exercise should be encouraged.
- *First-line* treatment involves NSAIDs.
  - Tylenol does not decrease inflammation, but that does not matter in this case. It may be a better choice because it avoids the issue of the side effects of long-term NSAID use.
- *Second-line*: steroid injections.
- *Third-line*: **glucosamine chondroitin** and **hyaluronic acid** injections (third line).
- *Fourth-line*: joint replacement surgery will be required if all other interventions fail.

Gout

Acute monoarticular arthritis caused by the deposit of "sodium urate crystals" in the intra-articular space.

Risk factors: dehydration (*most common*), hemolysis (cell turnover), chemotherapy, tumor lysis, alcohol, high red meat consumption, starvation, use of diuretics (loop diuretics and thiazides), and Lesch-Nyhan syndrome.

Hx/PE: The metatarsal-phalangeal joint of the great toe (podagra) is the most commonly affected joint. Patients may present with **tophi** (urate crystals in soft tissue) or **podagra** (uric acid in first MTP joint). Sudden excruciating joint pain, edema, and inflammation.

Diagnosis:

- CBC: elevated WBC count.
- Serum uric acid level (usually >7.5 mg/dL).
- Joint radiography: punched-out erosions—"rat bite."
- *Most accurate test*: diagnostic arthrocentesis "needle-shaped crystals" and strong "negative birefringence" under polarized light.

Treatment:

- Acute gout:
  - For *acute* gout, the *best initial treatment* is therapy with NSAIDs; these may be contraindicated in cases of acute renal failure.
  - Prednisone (oral [multiple joints] or injected) can be used in *acute* joint gout (but is not the first-line treatment because of the adverse side effects).
  - Colchicine and steroids (*second line*). Colchicine is not contraindicated in renal failure.
  - If a patient has acute renal failure, use corticosteroids or colchicine.

- Long-term treatment:
  - Dietary modification and allopurinol are used for *long-term treatment*.
  - Use allopurinol as prophylaxis if patients experience >3 attacks/year.
  - Never use probenecid, which is now rarely prescribed, and not the appropriate treatment.

- Prevention:
  - Treatment includes increased H_2O intake, weight loss, decreased consumption of red meats, and decreased alcohol intake.
  - Need to evaluate medications since thiazides and diuretics (loop diuretics) can cause increase in uric acid level (ACEi might be a better alternative in these cases).

Pseudogout

May involve calcification of articular cartilage, i.e., "calcium pyrophosphate dehydrate" crystal deposition.

Risk factors: elevated levels of parathyroid hormone (PTH) and calcium, hypothyroidism, and hemochromatosis.

Hx/PE: Usually involves larger joints, as opposed to gout.

Diagnosis: CBC, ionized calcium, PTH, bone radiography, and diagnostic arthrocentesis (shows "positive birefringence crystals" or **rhomboid crystals**).

Treatment:

- *Best initial treatment*: NSAIDs or steroids.
- Colchicine can prevent recurrent attacks.

Gonococcal arthritis

Migratory arthralgia and necrotic pustules can be seen.

Diagnosis: The *most accurate test* is arthrocentesis: Gram stain (to confirm presence of Gram-negative diplococci).

Treatment: IV or IM ceftriaxone.

Lumbosacral

Lumbosacral muscle strain or sprain

Strains and sprains are commonly caused by trauma. Patient usually has a stressor prior to the onset of pain.

Hx/PE: Pain reproducible on palpation of muscle or soft tissue (pain not directly on spine itself).

Diagnosis:

- Clinical diagnosis: pain on palpation of the muscle lateral to the spinal column.
- No imaging studies (spinal CT-scan or spinal MRI) are indicated in acute management of new-onset, muscular pain, or absence of neurologic signs.

Note: with muscle strain or sprain, if there is no improvement within 4 weeks or neurological focal signs; then perform a spinal MRI scan.

- Conservative management if mild/moderate pain: "RICE" (rest [initially], ice, compression, and exercise as tolerated). Continued activity, as tolerable, is recommended.
- In cases of severe pain: absolute bed rest.
- In cases of positive neurologic findings <u>or</u> positive straight leg test; then high-dose steroids are appropriate, followed by radiological studies.
- In case of cauda equina syndrome, immediate IV steroids, spinal MRI, and refer to a neurosurgeon or orthopedic surgeon immediately.

Lumbar disk herniation

Commonly caused by trauma or degenerative changes. Can progress to cauda equine syndrome.

Hx/PE: <u>Sudden</u> severe back pain, "electric-like" pain exacerbated by cough, defecation, and sneezing. Pain is common in L4-L5 or L5-S1. Positive straight leg test and hyperreflexia.

Diagnosis:

- Spinal radiography (*diagnostic*). ESR (to rule out infection). Alkaline phosphates and PSA (if metastasis is suspected).
- DEXA body scanning (<2.5), if osteoporosis is suspected.
- Stat spinal MRI if cauda equine syndrome is suspected.

Treatment:

- NSAIDs (scheduled dose) and/or analgesics depending on pain scale.
- Absolute bed rest for the first 1 to 2 days.
- Physical therapy (activity limitation) and local heat.
- The condition resolves in 4 weeks in 80% of patients.
- In case of cauda equine syndrome, surgical **discectomy** will be required.

Vertebral compression fracture

Common among elderly patients with osteoporosis or metastasis. Compression fractures can occur secondary to minor trauma in these populations. Spontaneous resolution is common.

Hx/PE: Sudden severe back pain with positive straight leg test.

Diagnosis:
- Spinal radiography (*first test*), ESR (to check for infections), and DEXA scan (to rule out osteoporosis).
- Alkaline phosphate, PSA levels, or mammogram (if metastasis is suspected).
- Spinal MRI (*specific*).

Treatment:
- *Most urgent step* is to give high-dose steroids (to help alleviate swelling).
- If the compression is caused by osteoporosis: give vitamin D, calcium supplementation, and encourage increased exercise.
- Surgical decompression would be required for sphincter defects, perineal anesthesia, or patients showing no resolution with conservative measures.

Lumbar spinal stenosis

Chronic narrowing of the lumbar or cervical spinal canal leading to compression of the nerve roots. Often associated with degenerative joint disease and is common in middle-aged and elderly patients.

Hx/PE: Lower back pain radiating to the buttocks, thighs, or legs. Leg numbness, weakness, and pain that improves with leaning forward and flexion of the spine. Romberg's test may show positive results.

Diagnosis:
- Spinal radiography: check for degenerative changes.
- Spinal MRI: *most specific diagnostic test.*
- DEXA scan: rule out osteoporosis.

Treatment:

- *First line therapy*: NSAIDs and physical therapy (abdominal muscle strengthening).
- Epidural corticosteroid injections (provide *short-term* relief).
- If the above treatments fail and progressive neurologic deficits or bladder dysfunction develops, surgical decompression (**laminectomy**) may be required.

Cauda equina syndrome

Surgical emergency

Spinal cord compression syndrome is commonly associated with prostate, breast, or lung cancer metastases.

Hx/PE: Sensory loss is usually <u>bilateral</u> which is different from the unilateral loss experienced in a stroke. Lower back pain, "saddle sensory disruption," and bowel and bladder dysfunction.

Diagnosis:

- Stat spinal MRI and IV high-dose steroids (emergency means treatment first).
- Ruling out of secondary causes such as metastasis (alkaline phosphates, PSA, mammograms, and rectal exams).

Treatment: IV high-dose steroids and emergency neurosurgery (**discectomy**).

Scoliosis

Defined as a lateral curvature of the spine of >10°, commonly in thoracic and/or lumbar spine. Rotation can be kyphosis or lordosis that is usually idiopathic. If the curvature is >60° with respiratory complaints, the patient should undergo a pulmonary function test and surgery must be considered.

Hx/PE: Back pain that improves with rest and usually observed on routine examination.

- Physical exam: Adam test (good screening test).
- Spinal radiography (best for precise evaluation): posterior, anterior, and full-length view.

Treatment:

- Curvature of <20°: observation.
- Curvature of 20–49°: spinal bracing.
- Curvature of >50°: surgical correction.

Upper extremity fractures and dislocations

<u>Techniques</u>:

➤ Closed reduction, if not badly displaced.

➤ Open reduction, if severely displaced.

➤ Keep in mind tetanus prevention and antibiotic prophylaxis in cases of open fractures.

➤ At least 2 view radiography, encompassing the joints above and below the fracture, is always required.

Shoulder anterior dislocation

Most common upper extremity dislocation, where the arm is slightly abducted and externally rotated and the forearm is rotated outward as if preparing to "shake hands." The nerves, tendons, and vessels need to be checked for signs of damage.

Diagnosis:

- *Best initial test*: shoulder radiography.
- *Most accurate test*: shoulder MRI especially if nerve damage is suspected.
- Angiogram, if vessel injury is suspected.

Treatment: Close reduction followed by sling and swathe.

Note: rule out axillary nerve injury.

Shoulder posterior dislocation

Common after a seizure, where the arm is adducted and internally rotated.

Diagnosis:

- *Best initial test*: shoulder radiography.
- *Most accurate test*: shoulder MRI especially if nerve damage is suspected.
- Angiogram, if vessel injury is suspected.

Treatment: Close reduction followed by sling and swathe.

Note: rule out radial artery injury.

Clavicular fracture

Clavicular fractures are usually caused by trauma.

Hx/PE: Pain over clavicle and possible symptoms of brachial plexus injury.

Diagnosis: *Best initial test* is clavicular radiography.

Treatment:

- Non-displaced fractures can usually be managed by conservative therapy (**simple arm sling**).
- Displaced clavicular fractures usually require open reduction and internal fixation.

Note:

- ✓ The figure eight sling for clavicular fractures are no longer used because its outcome is no better than that of the simple arm sling.
- ✓ Displaced fractures usually require open reduction and internal fixation.

Adhesive capsulitis (frozen shoulder)

Patient presents with shoulder immobility. Pain is usually worse at night. Patient usually with recent shoulder surgery. If develops chronic inflammation can cause fibrosis and contractures.

Hx/PE: Loss of active and passive motion in ≥ 2 planes. Pain is usually worse at night.

Diagnosis: Shoulder radiography (not always required but used to rule out other etiologies).

Note: nerve conduction studies and angiogram can be performed, if nerve or vasculature damage is suspected.

Treatment:
- Frequently self-limited and complete recovery in about 12 months.
- Hanging arm cast (rest) followed by physical therapy (gentle range of motion exercises).
- If conservative management fails (after ≥ 3 months), consider glucocorticoid injections.
- *Last resort* is surgery (after months to year).

Nightstick fracture

Ulnar shaft fracture usually resulting from self-defense.

Hx/PE: "Claw hand."

Diagnosis: Forearm radiography.

Note: nerve conduction studies and angiogram can be performed, if nerve or vasculature damage is suspected.

Treatment:
- Open reduction and internal fixation in cases of significant displacement.
- After open or closed reduction, a long arm cast can be applied.

Note: with casting, patients need to be monitored for compartment syndrome.

Boxer's fracture

A fracture involving the fourth or fifth metacarpal neck. Can be caused by closed fist boxing or fighting.

Diagnosis: Hand radiography.

Treatment:

- Closed reduction and **ulnar gutter splint**.
- If external lesions are present, amoxicillin plus clavulanic acid will be required. Tetanus vaccination must be administered, if applicable.

Note: any lacerations caused by a fist fight need to be monitored for infection with *Eikenella corrodens* (natural flora in humans).

Scaphoid fracture

Caused by falling on an outstretched hand. The carpal bone is the *most commonly* fractured bone in this case.

Hx/PE: Tenderness in the anatomical snuff box.

Diagnosis:

- Hand radiography scans may not show the fracture for 2 weeks.
- Hand bone scan takes about 3-5 days to show fracture.
- Hand MRI (immediate assessment) will show the fracture.

Treatment:

- Nondisplaced fracture: **thumb spica cast** regardless of radiographic findings.
- Displaced fracture: orthopedic surgeon referral.

Note: scaphoid fractures if not treated, can cause avascular necrosis.

Colles' fracture

Involves the <u>distal</u> radius from an "outstretched hand" and is referred to as a "dinner fork" deformity; more common among children and elderly patients.

Diagnosis: Forearm radiography.

Treatment: Open reduction, internal fixation surgery, and forearm cast.

Monteggia fracture

Proximal ulnar fracture with subluxation of the radial head.

Diagnosis: Elbow and forearm radiography (2 view).

Treatment:

- Open reduction and internal fixation of the ulnar and closed reduction of the radial head.
- Long-arm cast.

Galeazzi fracture

Diaphysis fracture of the distal radius and distal radioulnar joint.

Diagnosis: Wrist radiography.

Treatment: Open reduction and internal fixation; casting forearm in the supination position.

Dupuytren's contracture

Disease involving the palmar fascia, resulting in shortening and thickening of the fibrous bands in the hands and fingers.

Hx/PE: <u>Palpable</u> nodules and inability to extend fingers and place the hands flat on a table.

Diagnosis: Clinical diagnosis.

Treatment: Needle therapy and occasionally surgery.

Carpal tunnel syndrome

Entrapment neuropathy of the median nerve as it passes through the carpal tunnel of the wrist and compression of the median nerve. No studies have shown clear association with repetitive movement (overuse), however, can exacerbate symptoms.

Hx/PE: Pain on the radial three digits, tingling sensation, weakness, and pain exacerbation at nighttime. Can be associated with hypothyroidism, diabetes, RA, sarcoidosis, and pregnancy.

Diagnosis:

- *Best initial test* (clinical diagnosis):
  - Phalen's test (flexion of the wrist for 1 minute).
  - Tinel's test (tapping over the median nerve causes tingling) is more sensitive than Phalen's test.
- EMG and nerve conduction studies (*specific tests*).

Treatment:

- Wrist splint and rest for 2 to 6 weeks (*first-line treatment*).
- NSAIDs can be added to adjunctive therapy but not used as first-line treatment.
- If conservative treatment fails or thenar atrophy develops, administer steroid injections.
- Carpal tunnel release surgery (*most effective*) can be the *last resort*.

Lower extremity fractures and dislocations

Posterior hip dislocation

Orthopedic emergency

Risk factors: sciatic nerve injury and avascular necrosis (AVN).

Hx/PE: Commonly caused by "dashboard injury." Hip internally rotated, adducted, and flexed

Diagnosis: Hip radiography followed by hip CT scan after reduction.

Treatment: Emergency reduction (to avoid AVN) followed by **abduction pillow bracing**.

Note: be mindful of the likelihood of femoral AVN.

Anterior hip dislocation

Risk factor: obturator nerve damage.

Hx/PE: Hip externally rotated and abducted.

Diagnosis: Hip radiography followed by hip CT scan after reduction.

Treatment: Closed reduction followed by abduction pillow bracing.

Note: need to rule out femoral AVN. Angiograms might be needed in cases of severe pain, numbness, or tingling.

Hip fracture

The risk of fat embolism is very high in the first few days. Patients may develop AVN and DVTs.

Risk factors: advanced age, trauma, and osteoporosis.

Hx/PE: Fractures involving displacement of the femoral neck and shortened and externally rotated leg.

Diagnosis: Hip radiography and hip MRI. Rule out osteoporosis with DEXA scan.

Treatment:

- Open reduction and internal fixation with parallel pinning of the femoral neck. Surgery can be delayed when necessary but best results are when surgery is prompt.

  - Advanced age is not usually a contrindication for surgery.

- Elderly patients will require **hemiarthroplasty** (replacement of the native bone with a metal prosthesis) and DVT prophylaxis.

- LMWH is prophylactic therapy; however, LMWH will need to be stopped 12 hours before surgery.

Note: hip replacement will be required if the acetabulum and femoral head have been displaced.

Femoral fracture

Most commonly caused by trauma. Patients can develop anemia, secondary to blood loss. Need to be aware of the likelihood of fat emboli (presents with hypoxia, tachycardia, tachypnea, and altered mental status). On physical examination, always rule out vascular problems.

Diagnosis: CBC (to detect anemia), femoral radiography (*diagnostic*), and femoral MRI scan (to detect osteonecrosis).

Treatment:

- Open reduction and internal fixation with intramedullary nailing of the femur or hemiarthroplasty.

- Total hip replacement is the treatment of choice for stage 4 osteonecrosis.

- LMWH can be used for prophylactic therapy to prevent DVT.

Preventions:

- ➢ Elderly patients may benefit from a home evaluation assessment and "**get up and go**" test.

- ➢ Consider early immobilization and operative fixation of the fracture to prevent fat embolism.

Note: the risk of fat embolism is reduced with the passage of time after the fracture.

Tibial fracture

Direct trauma to the low extremity and high risk of **compartment syndrome**.

Diagnosis:
- Tibial radiography (*diagnostic*).
- Relieving compartmental pressure, if compartment syndrome develops.

Treatment: Casting or intramedullary nailing.

Stress fracture

Usually caused by playing competitive sports.

Diagnosis:
- Radiography (may not show fracture).
- Bone scan (will show increased uptake).

Treatment: Rest, NSAIDs, and possible casting/bracing.

Note: these fractures takes about 4 to 6 weeks to heal.

Morton neuroma

Inflammation of the common digital nerve (between the third and fourth toes) of the third interspace caused by wearing high heels and pointed-toe shoes.

Diagnosis: Clinical diagnosis and palpable neuroma.

Treatment: Analgesics and comfortable footwear.

Upper extremity nerves and tendons

Trigeminal neuralgia (tic douloureux)

Hx/PE: Unilateral, severe, stabbing, and electric pain along the trigeminal nerve.

Diagnosis:

- Clinical diagnosis: neurological exam.
- Head MRI to rule out MS.

Treatment: The treatment of choice is therapy with carbamazepine.

Note: need to get baseline CBC (WBC) lbefore treatment with carbamazepine..

Brachial plexus injury

Common injury after clavicular fracture.

Hx/PE: Generalized weakness and loss of sensation in the entire upper extremity.

Diagnosis: Cervical radiography, EMG (in case of nerve damage), nerve conduction studies (in case of nerve damage), and angiogram (if vascular damage is suspected).

Treatment: Surgery.

Subacromial bursitis

Pain when the arm is actively raised laterally above the head. Usually no pain at rest.

De Quervain's tenosynovitis

Mothers who support their infants' head with a hyperextended thumb and flexed wrist.

Diagnosis: Clinical diagnosis (Finkelstein's test).

Treatment: Rest, NSAIDs, and steroid injections.

Common nerve damage post-surgery

➤ Mastectomy surgery can cause damage to the long thoracic nerve.

➤ Mandible surgery can cause damage to the hypoglossal nerve.

➤ Parathyroid surgery can cause damage to the facial nerve.

Long thoracic nerve injury

Damage can be caused by the use of crutches or injury to the lateral part of the ribs, resulting in a "winged scapula." Common after breast surgery.

Axillary nerve injury

Affects the nerve innervating the deltoid muscles and compensates the ability to abduct the shoulder. Common after shoulder dislocation or anterior shoulder dislocation.

Radial nerve injury

The radial nerve innervates the triceps, brachioradialis, supinator of the forearm, and extensors of the wrist. Injury to the nerve is termed as "wrist drop"; and can be caused by humeral fracture.

Lower extremity ligaments and nerves

Anterior cruciate ligament injury

Caused by forced hyperextension of the knee or by impact. Can cause rapid hemarthrosis (blood in joint fluid).

Diagnosis: Clinical diagnosis (**positive anterior drawer test**) and knee MRI (*specific*).

Treatment:

- Physical therapy and pain control (NSAIDs).
- **Arthroscopic surgery** with a graft from the patellar or hamstring tendon.

Note: patellar tendon tear can cause excruciating pain, difficulty bearing weight, and swelling.

Posterior cruciate ligament injury

Caused by forced hyperextension or trauma, such as "dash board injury."

Diagnosis: Clinical diagnosis (**positive posterior drawer test**) and knee MRI (*specific*).

Treatment:

- Physical therapy and pain control (NSAIDs).
- Arthroscopic surgery is usually considered for highly competitive athletes.

Meniscal injury

Twisting injury or degenerative tear and <u>not</u> associated with hemarthrosis.

Hx/PE: Popping sound heard during flexion and extension of the knee.

Diagnosis:

- Positive McMurray maneuver: used to evaluate the lateral and medial meniscus.
  - Internal rotation: pain and popping sound, indicating tear in the lateral meniscus.
  - External rotation: pain and popping sound, indicating tear in the medial meniscus.
- Knee MRI (*specific*).

Treatment:

- Physical therapy: *first-line treatment*.
- NSAIDs: pain management.
- Arthroscopic evaluation and intervention are necessary when conservative management fails.

Post-total knee replacement

Patients must be administered therapy with anticoagulants, e.g., LMWH or warfarin, as they are at a high risk of DVT caused by immobility.

Achilles tendon rupture

Usually occurs in middle-age patients with decreased exercise conditioning or patients on fluoroquinolones.

Hx/PE: A pop like a "rifle shot" can be expressed by patients. Board exams usually give an example of a person playing tennis.

Diagnosis: Thompson test (pressure on the gastrocnemius leading to absence of foot plantar flexion).

Treatment: Surgical repair followed by long leg cast for 6 weeks.

Note:

✓ Patients with Achilles tendon rupture must <u>never</u> be given a steroid injection.

✓ Patients on long term quinolones need to be aware of risk factor of tendon ruptures.

Piriformis syndrome

Compression of the sciatic nerve as it exits the <u>greater</u> sciatic foramen below the piriformis muscle. Pain is worsened during sitting and patients describe the symptoms as a tingling and aching sensation.

Tarsal tunnel syndrome

Tenosynovitis inflammation is similar to carpal tunnel syndrome but with <u>tibial nerve</u> involvement.

Hx/PE: Pain is aggravated with increased use.

Treatment: Rest, NSAIDs (*first-line*), steroid injections, and surgical release may be required if conservative treatment fails.

Femoral nerve injury

Loss of the ability to extend knee, loss of sensation over anterior and medial thigh, medial shin, and arch of foot.

Obturator nerve injury

Weakness in leg adduction and sensory loss over a smaller area of the medial thigh (comparted to femoral nerve). Can be damaged during pelvic trauma.

Fibromyalgia

Centrally mediated chronic pain, usually in the soft tissue and axial skeletal tissues and <u>absence</u> of joint pain. Common in women aged 30 to 50 years and associated with depression, anxiety, IBS, and others.

Hx/PE: Multiple tender points with at least 11 out of 18 pre-defined tender points of physical examination. If <11 tender points, it is known as myofascial pain syndrome.

Diagnosis: CPK, ANA, aldolase, ESR, TSH, and CBC (for differential diagnosis).

Treatment:

- *Initial treatment* is exercise and therapy with pregabalin (*best initial medication*), low-dose TCAs (more side effects), or muscle relaxants.
- Physical therapy and cognitive behavioral therapy are helpful.

Note: avoid narcotics and NSAIDs with fibromyalgia.

Muscle-related autoimmune and inflammation disorders

Costochondritis

Inflammation of the area where the ribs connect with the cartilage of the sternum.

Hx/PE: Localized chest pain reproduced when the cartilage is pressed.

Diagnosis:

- Differential diagnosis.
- Rule out other pathologies (GERD, MI, angina, pneumonia, and pancreatitis).

Treatment: Usually self-resolved. NSAIDs can be prescribed if no contraindications.

Polymyalgia rheumatica

Usually observed in females aged over 50 years.

Risk factors: this condition is often associated with **temporal arteritis**.

Hx/PE: Constitutional symptoms: fever, malaise, and weight loss. Inability to brush one's hair or climb stairs, severe muscle pain, stiffness in the shoulder and pelvic girdle, and <u>mild</u> weakness. Patients complain of pain more often than of weakness.

Diagnosis:
- Primarily a clinical diagnosis and elevated ESR [> 60 mm/h] can be used for confirmation.
- Normal levels of ANA, CPK, aldolase, and anti-Jo-1.

Treatment: Low-dose prednisone.

Polymyositis

A progressive, systemic disease caused by immune-mediated striated muscle inflammation, commonly involves proximal muscle weakness.

Hx/PE: Inability to get up from a chair, comb hair, and climb up a staircase. Difficulty in swallowing and breathing and muscle <u>weakness</u> and pain.

Diagnosis:
- *Initial tests*: CPK, aldolase, ANA, and anti-Jo-1 (increased levels).
- EMG (*specific*).
- The *most accurate test*: muscle biopsy (showing inflammation of muscle fibers and varying stages of necrosis and regeneration).

Treatment:
- High-dose corticosteroids that can be tapered after about a month.
- Can switch to azathioprine and/or MTX.

Dermatomyositis

Autoimmune disease that is more common in females. Can have risk of developing cancers (ovarian, lung, or colorectal cancer).

Hx/PE: Can present with heliotrope erythema, gottron papules, proximal muscle weakness, and rashes.

Diagnosis:

- *Initial tests*: CPK, aldolase, anti-Jo-1 (associated with interstitial lung disease), and ANA.
- EMG must be performed before muscle biopsy (neither test is an initial test).
- Muscle biopsy can be performed for a *definitive diagnosis* (but not always needed).
- Ovarian and colorectal cancer must be ruled out (chest, abdominal, and pelvic CT scan).

Treatment: Prednisone that can be tapered and later switched with azathioprine and/or MTX.

Note: azathioprine purine analog is converted to 6-mercaptopurine (6MP).

Scleroderma

Systemic sclerosis characterized by fibrosis and inflammation and abnormal deposition of collagen (type I and type III) in the body. Can cause GERD by decreasing esophageal peristalsis and lower esophageal sphincter pressure, where a chronic condition can lead to Barrett's esophagus.

Hx/PE:

- ➤ CREST syndrome (limited form): "CREST" calcinosis, Raynaud's phenomenon, esophageal dysfunction, sclerodactyly, and telangiectasia. No heart, lung, or kidney involvement.
- ➤ Diffuse scleroderma: can occur in various parts of the body including the organs. Dysphagia, thick skin, and cold extremities.

Diagnosis: RF (positive), ANA (positive in 95% of cases), **anti-centromere antibodies** (CREST syndrome), and **anti-topoisomerase (anti-Scl 70)**.

Treatment: Treat underlying symptoms:

- Acute flares: steroids (*first-line therapy*).
- Skin changes: penicillamine.
- Raynaud's phenomenon: calcium channel blockers (nifedipine).
- Hypertension and renal involvement: ACE inhibitors.
- GERD: high-dose proton-pump inhibitors (often for life).

Note: most common cause of death is pulmonary hypertension (caused by lung fibrosis).

Raynaud phenomenon: blue to purple discoloration of distal extremities (fingers and toes) when exposed to cold caused by arterial vasospasm.

Systemic Lupus Erythematosus (SLE)

Multisystem autoimmune disorder more common among females and African-Americans.

Hx/PE: Non-specific symptoms such as fever, weight loss, increased frequency of infections, and symmetric joint pain.

"**IM DARN SHARP**" elevated Igg levels, malar rash, discoid rash, arthritis, renal problems, neurologic symptoms, serositis, hematological abnormalities, ANA, RA (no joint destruction), and photosensitivity.

Four symptoms must be present, including positivity for ANA and anti-dsDNA, for a definitive diagnosis.

Diagnosis:
- ANA test (*best screening test*).
- **Anti-SM antibody** (*most specific*) and **anti-dsDNA** (can be used to follow disease).
- Drug-induced lupus (**anti-histone antibodies**); if negative results are obtained, the condition may not be associated with medication.
    - ANA test is a good way to rule out drug induced lupus.
- Neonatal SLE: **anti-Ro antibodies** (risk of heart block).
- PTT (mildly elevated).

- Joint radiography (no signs of joint destruction).
- CBC (anemia of chronic diseases, leukopenia, and/or thrombocytopenia).
- Urinalysis (possible proteinuria in later stages).
- If SLE nephritis is suspected, a renal biopsy must be performed to determine the staging and treatment plan.
- Almost 50% of the patients with lupus flares tend to have <u>low</u> complement levels (C3 and C4).

Note: patients with **drug-induced lupus** do <u>not</u> present with CNS or renal involvement and will have normal anti-dsDNA and complement levels. Keep in mind ANA and anti-histone antibodies can be positive.

Treatment:
- NSAIDs (for joint pain).
- Corticosteroids (for *acute* exacerbations).
    - Dosage depends on the severity of the disease.
- Hydroxychloroquine (usually used for *milder* disease) cyclophosphamide (used for more *severe* disease), and azathioprine (*long-term* control).
- Indications of steroids: renal involvement, thrombocytopenia, hemolytic anemia, CNS involvement, and SLE pericarditis.
- **Anti-phospholipid antibody syndrome**: needs to be treated with heparin if **pregnant** and warfarin if not pregnant.
- Sunblock use, rheumatology consultation (if needed), and nephrology consultation (if needed).
- **Neonatal lupus** can be associated with risk of complete heart block caused by the circulating antibodies.

Possible side effects of steroid use:
- Diabetes, hypertension, thinning of the skin, psychosis, myopathy, hyperglycemia, acne, immune system impairment, candida, cataracts, glaucoma, and osteoporosis.
- Steroid-induced psychosis (dose needs to be tapered).
- All patients on steroids should be placed on PPIs or anti-histamine blockers for prophylaxis.
- Patients on chronic steroids should undergo DEXA scanning

(to rule out osteoporosis) and be placed on vitamin D and calcium prophylaxis.

- **Avascular necrosis (AVN)** especially in the femoral head. Present with dull pain during leg movement and decreased range of motion.
  - MRI (the *best test* for detecting early AVN, which can be seen on radiographic scans in the advanced stages).

Anti-phospholipid antibody syndrome

Can occur independent of SLE. Increases risk of spontaneous abortions.

Hx/PE: Hypercoagulability.

Diagnosis:
- ANA antibody can be helpful for detecting anti-phospholipid antibody syndrome.
- Pregnant patients need to be screened for anti-Ro and anti-La antibody.
- **Anti-cardiolipin antibody** (*sensitive* test).

Treatment:
- *Life-long* warfarin with target INR between 2.0 and 3.0.
- Warfarin must be switched with low molecular weight heparin in case of pregnant patients.

Sjogren's syndrome

Autoimmune inflammatory disease characterized by lymphocytic infiltration of the salivary and lacrimal glands, causing decreased production of tears and saliva. Patients are at a <u>risk</u> of developing NHL.

Hx/PE: Xerostomia, dry eyes, itchy eyes "sandy" feeling under the eyelids, difficulty in swallowing food, dental loss, and vaginal dryness.

Diagnosis:
- Schirmer's test (a dry paper is placed in the lower eyelid pouch and decreased moistening of the paper can help diagnose keratoconjunctivitis sicca).

- Anti-Ro/SSA and anti-La/SSB (positive).
- ANA test and RF tests (to rule out autoimmune disease like SLE [most common association] and RA).
- *Most accurate test*: biopsy of the salivary glands of the lip (more sensitive than the anti-Ro and anti-La test).

Treatment:
- Keep the eye moist with artificial tears to avoid further corneal damage and use of vaginal lubrication.
- Pilocarpine (to increase oral and ocular secretions).

Ankylosing spondylitis

Chronic inflammation of spine and pelvis that leads to sacroiliitis and fusion of the affected joints; age of onset is usually early 20s.

Common presentation: male gender, family history, aortic insufficiency, anterior uveitis, restrictive lung disease, and heart block. Uveitis is the *most common* complication occurring in about 30–40% of the patients.

Other forms of spondylitis must be ruled out:

➤ Reactive arthritis (Reiter's syndrome): associated with a history of GI (*shigella, Salmonella*, or *campylobacter*) or GU infections caused by infection with *Chlamydia trachomatis*. Reactive arthritis secondary to chlamydia is more common in the presents of HLA-B27. Patients present with arthritis, urethritis, uveitis, and conjunctivitis: "can't see, pee, or climb a tree."

- Treatment: NSAIDs.

➤ Psoriatic arthritis: involves both PIP and DIP joints, distal destruction, asymmetric arthritis, nail changes (pitting) occur in 85%, "sausage-shaped" digits (dactylitis), and psoriatic skin changes.

- Treatment: NSAIDs and/or MTX (if resistant).

➤ Enteropathic spondylitis: ankylosing spondylitis-like condition associated with inflammatory bowel disease.

Hx/PE: Lower back pain that "improves with movement," decreased spine flexion (Schober's test), hip pain, and stiffness.

Overall diagnosis:

- *Best initial test*: spinal radiography of fused sacroiliac joints ("**bamboo spine**"). The scans may not show such changes at early onset.

- *Most accurate test*: spinal MRI (can help visualize the pathology at early stages).

- HLA-B27 (positive), echocardiogram (aortic regurgitation), ESR (elevated), ANA (negative), and RF (negative).

Note:

✓ Monitor disease progression every 3 months with spinal radiography and ESR.

✓ Also note there is <u>no</u> decreased in life expectancy in these patients.

Overall treatment:

- *First-line therapy*: physical therapy, exercise (helps improve flexibility and posture), TNF inhibitors, and NSAIDs.

- Sulfasalazine (refractory cases).

- *Oral steroids are <u>not</u> helpful.

Giant cell arteritis

Subacute *granulomatous inflammation* of the large vessels including the aorta, internal carotid, and temporal branch.

<u>Risk</u> of developing **polymyalgia rheumatica** (proximal muscle pain but <u>not</u> weakness).

Hx/PE: More common in elderly patients. Can cause blindness and secondary obstruction of internal carotid artery.

Diagnosis:

- Clinical examination <u>plus</u> elevated ESR.

- Even in cases of clinical suspicion, a complete physical exam is necessary before administering steroids.

- If symptoms are <u>not</u> relieved within 72 hours after initiation of therapy with steroids, perform temporal artery biopsy (*most accurate test*).

- Need to measure baseline DEXA scan values before giving high-dose steroids.

Treatment:
- In cases of visual changes and elevated ESR levels, immediate treatment with high-dose IV steroids will be necessary.
- Once the symptoms improve, low-dose steroid therapy can be maintained.
- Can monitor response by ESR levels.

Vascular

Subclavian steal syndrome

Hx/PE: Vascular symptoms manifesting as cold, tingling, and muscle pain in the upper extremities usually during exercise involving the upper extremities.

Diagnosis: Upper extremity Doppler sonography and angiogram.

Treatment: Balloon angioplasty, stenting, and bypass surgery.

Churg-Strauss syndrome

A type of vasculitis, which occasionally arises in asthmatic and allergic rhinitis patients.

Hx/PE: Renal failure, palpable purpura, and respiratory symptoms.

Diagnosis:
- *Initial tests*: CBC (eosinophilia), UA, and BUN/Cr ratio.
- *Best screening test*: P-ANCA (elevated levels).
- *Most accurate test*: biopsy.

Treatment: Steroids (immunosuppressant's) and cyclophosphamide.

Note: P-ANCA is also associated with polyarteritis nodosa.

Polyarteritis nodosa (PAN)

Hx/PE: Rash, fever, weight gain, erythema nodosum, arthritis, and abdominal pain. Associated with HBV.

Diagnosis:

- *Initial tests*: CBC, UA, BUN/Cr ratio, and urine culture.
- *Best screening test*: P-ANCA and hepatic viral panel.
- *Most specific test*: renal biopsy.

Treatment: Immunosuppressant's (steroids and cyclophosphamide).

Pediatric orthopedics

Juvenile idiopathic arthritis

Also known as juvenile rheumatoid arthritis. Patient are usually aged below 16 years and show the symptoms for >6 weeks. Those positive for ANA have a good prognosis and patients with a rheumatoid factor (RF) positivity have a poor prognosis

Hx/PE: Morning stiffness and joint pain in patients aged <16 years, for at least 6 weeks.

- ➤ Pauciarticular: uveitis/blindness (slit lamp), involvement of <5 joints, and no systemic symptoms.
    - Diagnosis: +ANA, –RF, and joint radiography.
- ➤ Polyarthritis: mild disease, involvement of >5 joints, and no systemic symptoms.
    - Diagnosis: +ANA, –RF, and joint radiography.
- ➤ Still's disease: salmon colored macular rash, involvement of >5 joints, and fever (body temperature, >39°C).
    - Diagnosis: +ANA, –RF, and joint radiography.

Treatment:

- NSAIDs (*first line*).
- MTX (*second line*) and steroids (*acute*).
- Carditis: steroids.

Note: folic acid to be given with MTX.

Developmental dysplasia of the hip

Femoral head has an abnormal relationship to the acetabulum. The risk of osteoarthritis increases in adulthood.

Hx/PE: Female gender, breach birth, family history, and first-born infants. Evaluate with Barlow test.

Diagnosis: Bilateral hip radiography.

Treatment:

- Treatment should be managed by an orthopedic surgeon.
- **Pavlik harness** is the *first line treatment* and most affective up to the age of 6 months.
- If the Pavlik harness is ineffective, then closed reduction can be performed, followed by a **spica cast**.
- If closed reduction fails, then perform open reduction.

Osteogenesis imperfecta

Autosomal dominant disease associated with abnormal collagen synthesis.

Hx/PE: Hearing loss, bone fractures, teeth abnormalities, and blue sclera.

Diagnosis:

- Genetic testing (*specific*).
- CBC, PTT, PT, bleeding time, and platelets (to rule out child abuse).

Duchenne muscular dystrophy

X-linked recessive disorder; *dystrophin* is located in the plasma membrane of muscle fibers owing to a mutation in the gene coding for the plasma membrane protein for the muscle fibers. In patients aged above 5 years, this disorder is called **Becker's muscular dystrophy**.

Hx/PE: Gluteal weakness, intellectual impairment, and "wobbly" gait.

Diagnosis:

- Genetic screening.
- CPK (usually elevated owing to muscle damage).
- Blood sample PCR for abnormal dystrophin protein.
- Muscle biopsy for *definitive* diagnosis.

Legg-Calve-Perthes disease

Idiopathic AVN of the femoral head and is common in young children. Patients usually aged between 3 and 5 years, presenting with hip pain and/or limp. Pain is worsened with activity and relieved with rest.

Note: AVN in the pediatric population can also be observed in patients with sickle cell disease and Legg-Calve-Perthes disease.

Diagnosis:

- Pelvic radiography (the scans could appear normal).
- Initial <u>wide</u> articular space and necrosis of the femoral head on MRI scan.

Treatment: Self-healing with the goal of maintaining joint mobility and stabilizing the hip in the acetabulum with bracing or casting.

Osgood-Schlatter disease

"Pain in the tibial tubercle" and patella after repetitive exercise. Usually active children aged 10–15 years.

Hx/PE: Tenderness on palpation over the tibial tubercle, soft-tissue swelling, and prominence of the tubercle. Range of motion is usually normal.

Diagnosis: Knee radiography and clinical examination.

Treatment:

- Cases of mild disease can be treated with rest, bracing, and icing.
- Continued physical activity is encouraged.

X-linked hypophosphatemic rickets

X-linked; characterized by hypophosphatemia and rickets.

Hx/PE: Urine excretion of phosphate is abnormally high.

Diagnosis:

- Genetic testing.
- All common electrolytes are at normal levels except for phosphate, which is low.
- Normal serum calcium, normal to high PTH, increased alkaline phosphatase, and normal to low 1,25-dihydroxycholecalciferol.

Slipped capital-femoral epiphysis

Medical emergency

Overweight children/teens aged 9 to 13 years.

Hx/PE: Severe pain, external rotational deformity, inability to rotate leg internally, limb shortening, and inability to bear weight. Typically, the patients are obese with delayed skeletal maturation and recent growth spurt.

Diagnosis: Bilateral lateral films and AP films.

Treatment: No weight bearing, rest, and immediate internal fixation (stabilization with screws).

Familial short stature (genetic short stature)

Commonly present with normal length and weight at birth until about 3 years of age. After 3 years of age, the growth and weight begins to decline. They have normal puberty onset and a decline in height by more than 2 standard deviations below the mean.

Diagnosis:

- Shorter than normal teens compare **bone age to chronologic age**.
- Rule out secondary causes: TSH, FSH, LH, GnRH, testosterone, estrogen, genetic screening, and GH levels.

Growing pain

Growing pains usually occur at the age of 5 and 11 years. Usually bilateral deep pain. Work-up would be negative. Rule out RA and bone tumors.

Hx/PE: Deep bone pain that is usually bilateral and worse at night.

Diagnosis: Clinical diagnosis and further work-up not required.

Treatment: Massage and NSAIDs.

Index

Index, cont'd.

Hematology & Musculoskeletal In Your Pocket

Index, cont'd.

Index, cont'd.

splenic sequestration 20
splenic sequestration crises 19
Still's disease 73
stress fracture 58
subclavian steal syndrome 72
systemic lupus erythematosus 67

T

tarsal tunnel syndrome 63
tartrate-resistant acid
 phosphatase 30
terminal deoxynucleotidyl
 transferase 26
thalassemia 15
thrombotic thrombocytopenic
 purpura 10
thumb spica cast 53
tibial fracture 58
tic douloureux 59
Tinel's test 55
tissue plasminogen activator 7
tophi 44
transfusion allergic reaction 38
transplant rejection 39
transplants, types 39
trigeminal neuralgia 59
tumor lysis syndrome 31

U

ulnar gutter splint 53
upper extremity fractures 50
upper extremity nerves 59
uroporphyrinogen decarboxylase,
 25

V

vaso-occlusion crisis 20
vertebral compression fracture 48
viral induced thrombo-
 cytopenia 13
von Willebrand's disease 5

W

Waldenstrom's macroglobulinemia
 35
warfarin 6
warfarin-induced skin necrosis 7

X

X-linked hypophosphatemic rickets
 76

Hematology & Musculoskeletal In Your Pocket